# SECRETS OF

# CHILD TECHNOLOGY

## (CHILD BY PLANNING NOT BY CHANCE)



Shiv Ram Tiwari

(M. Sc) Retd. Scientist

KAVYA
PUBLICATIONS

**Publisher:**

**SDR INNOWAYS INDIA PVT. LTD.**
667, Rajaward, Kulpahar, Mahoba - 210426

Imprint:
**KAVYA PUBLICATIONS**
Abhinav R.H.4, Awadhpuri, Bhopal - 462002

**Centre**
Kavya Publications
(Maxel Electronics) 8, 3rd floor DSIDC Shed SCHEME-1
Okhla phase -2, Delhi - 20.

**Mob. :** 7905266820, 9918801353
**Website:** www.kavyapublications.com
**E-Mail:** editor@kavyapublications.com

**ISBN :** 978-93-6431-338-4
**Price :** 399/-
**Published Date :** 2025


This book is printed at MTL and published by Ajay Agrawal, CEO of SDR Innoways India Pvt. Ltd. Kulpahar Mahoba with its imprint and centre, Kavya Publications Delhi.

# PREFACE

Motive of this project is to give very new as well as noble concept regarding fertilization in human life science to get like child to balance the social system of living in the present world. This is a Noble work generated in my mind since very long time when I was married so early at the age of 16 in 1963 and was studying in High school. I have taken science & Biology as my subject to study the biological function in human life. Up to B.Sc., Biology & Chemistry was my pet subject and I have studied biological functions perfectly. But further more I did M.Sc. in Chemistry in 1971 from Lucknow University, Lucknow, UP India. With my perfection I have applied the biological function as an experiment with full precaution on my own life with the help of my wife and get 100% success in this field and get three male child one by one with full confidence of this concept.

I was very much anxious to know the 'Child Technology especially in human life to control population of the country and also to make balance of Male & Female gender difference in the social development of the society of the country. In this respect I have found a clue when I have studied many horoscopes of male and female child due to my interest in horoscopic study. I have found that there is surprising great difference in the horoscope of male & female child found hand written by the old Indian astrologers. In the horoscope of male child it was found mentioned that "Tasya Bharyam Daksh Kukshaw Utpanna" which means the child is born from the functioning of right ovary to produce ovum for fertilization to give birth of male child by that lady similarly in the horoscope of female child it was found mentioned that "Tasya Bharyam Vam Kukshaw Utpanna" which means the child is born from the functioning of left ovary to produce ovum for fertilization to give birth of female child by that lady.

The above said point is found very interesting to me for my project to have like child and for "CHILD-TECHNOLOGY" in human life. This provides me a way to have "CHILD BY PLANNING NOT BY CHANCE". Thus by performing FMT (Follicular Monitoring Test) after 8th day of M.C we can know the functioning of ovary and can get good result after insemination with taking required precautions.

The old Indian History certified that like child can be borne by applying this "CHILD TECHNOLOGY" with required precaution for eg. in Treta Yug Bhagwan Ram, Laxman,, Bharat, Satrughan and in Dwaper Yug

Yudhisthir, Arjun, Bhim, Nakul, Sahdev, even Karn will also born by this technology which is very much scientific in nature .

Objective of this project related to the "Selective Fertilization of gametes in Human" is very important and useful for the shake of society in its development.

It will protect the poverty, property dispute, educational burden of many child and population control by having one male and one female child only to full fill the social need of the society. It is also very useful in generation saving and balancing the gender ratio. Thus our statement is 100% true that- "Child by planning not by chance" "Ham do Hamare do one male and one female ho" by selective .

# ABSTRACT

The present work provides a method of reproduction by selective fertilization of gametes in humans. To plan a child in this method, the couple perform systematic intercourse near about the mid-point day of the menstrual cycle (MC), based on the status of the oviduct from HSG test and the required enlargement of the ovary and rupturing of the follicle based on Follicular Monitoring Test (FMT), and follow post intercourse actions in a guided manner. The intercourse is performed based on the desire of conceiving a female child or a male child, wherein an enlargement of the left side ovary and rupturing of the follicle with the systematic intercourse and post-intercourse procedure leads to the conception of a female child, and an enlargement of the right side ovary and rupturing of the follicle with the Systematic intercourse and post-intercourse procedure leads to the conception of a male child.

## DEFINITION

As used in the present work (except in the background art of the work), the following terms are generally intended to have the meaning as set forth below, except to the extent that the context in which they are used indicates otherwise.

As used herein, the terms "fallopian tube", "oviduct" may have been used interchangeably, and they mean the same. "Oviduct" or "fallopian tube" is the tube through which an ovum or egg passes from an ovary to the uterus in every MC.

As used herein, the terms "intercourse" or "sexual intercourse" means the penetration of penis of a man into the vagina of a woman repeatedly until the sperm from the man's penis ejaculates deep into the woman's vagina. The terms "intercourse" or "sexual intercourse" may have been used interchangeably, and they mean the same.

As used herein, the terms "sleeping" "sleep", "lying" or "lying down" may have been interchangeably used, which means a person lying on the bed with or without closing the eyes, with our without being awake.

As used herein, the term "couple" means a pair of "a man and a woman" possessing the legal age to have intercourse, and legally and ethically permitted to perform intercourse among themselves, and legally and ethically permitted to become parents of their child.

As used herein, the term "menstrual cycle" abbreviated form "MC" or "cycle" may have been interchangeably used. which means the periodical vaginal discharge of endometrial layer with blood happens to women of reproductive age.

# CONTENTS

# BACKGROUND OF THE WORK

According to existing reproductive process/ technology there is no certainty to get an offspring of a desired gender and it solely depends upon natural coincidence which provides unwanted results leading to population explosion, gender ratio imbalance, gender crimes, female foeticide, and discontinuation of ancestral chain and property disputes in the families resulting into huge pendency of civil suits in the courts.

It is known that, sperms are produced by the meiotic division of the male germinal cells present in the testes. This meiotic cell division results in the formation of two haploid cells containing 23 chromosomes (22 autosomes and 1 sex chromosome either x or y) from a diploid cell containing 23 pairs of chromosome in its nucleus (22 pairs of autosomes and 1 pair of sex chromosome x or y) One of this haploid cell results into a sperm containing 22 unpaired autosome and 1 unpaired 'X' chromosome and the other haploid cell results in to a sperm containing 22 unpaired autosome unpaired autosome and I unpaired 'Y' chromosome.

According to a report in WebMed By Dulce Zamora.

https://www.webmd.com/baby/features/choosing-sex-of- your-child#1)

In his book How to Choose the Sex of Your Baby, Shettles explains that the male (Y) sperm is smaller, faster, and more short-lived than the female (X) sperm. Because of this, it is better for boy-desiring couples to have sex closest to the time when a woman's egg is released (ovulation). This way, the speedy male sperm could get to the egg sooner than the female one.

The same article also in another paragraph says,

The Y chromosome apparently also enjoys an advantage over its counterpart when the sperm is discharged as close as possible to the opening of the **cervix**. This is achieved through rear entry intercourse (man enters woman from behind).

Parents desiring a girl, on the other hand, are encouraged to have sex in the missionary position (face to face, man on top) about two to four days before **ovulation** so that by the time the egg comes, only the heartier, more resilient X sperm will remain in the woman's reproductive tract.

According to an article madeformums in By Sarah Barker (https://www.madeformums.com/getting-pregnant/6- natural-ways-to-choose-your-babys-sex-and-their-success- rates/)

Dr. Landrum Shettles developed this theory in the US in the 1960s. It's complemented by the Billings Method, which is about timing sex around the consistency of vaginal mucus (when it's thin and clear for boys, thicker and stickier for girls). It's said that couples using this method tend to have boys more than girls.

Male sperm are more vulnerable and the vagina becomes less acidic closer to the cervix. So if penetration is deep (woman- on-top or man-behind positions), the male sperm will enter a more alkaline environment and are more likely to survive the short journey. Therefore, deeper positions should mean a boy is more likely.

Shallow penetration should favor your chances of conceiving a girl the slower female sperm are hard enough to withstand the acidic conditions at the entrance to the vagina so could make it through to the egg after the male sperm have died off.

Abstaining for a few days before making love increases your chances of conceiving a boy. The greater the volume of sperm, the more male sperm should be present, so theoretically there's a greater chance that a male sperm survives and fertilizes the egg before a female sperm can reach it.

The minerals in your diet could affect your metabolism and the environment of your eggs.

- To improve conditions for male sperm you need potassium (in meat, bananas, apricots and celery).

- To Improve conditions for female sperm you need more magnesium-rich food (in nuts, soya beans and leafy green vegetables).

If you reach orgasm before your partner, your vagina becomes more alkaline, which creates a better environment for male sperm. Female sperm survive better in the naturally acidic environment of your vagina, so climaxing first would favor the conception of boys.

Male sperm favor alkaline conditions, so douching (flooding the vagina via a syringe) with a dilute alkaline solution, such as sodium bicarbonate (baking soda) before intercourse increases the chances of conceiving a boy.

US6773726B2 discloses a method to take advantage of naturally occurring factors that influence gender selection *in* such a way as to create a bias to conceive a specific gender. This is accomplished by teaching a woman how to recognize the various stages of her menstrual cycle and how and when to use ovulation predictor reagent strips to accurately predict when ovulation will occur. Specific instructions are provided as to when a couple should engage in intercourse. The method for influencing the chances of conceiving a child of a selected gender includes the steps of following a selected diet; supplementing said diet with selected nutraceuticals; douching with a selected douche prior to intercourse; and selectively timing intercourse.

US6610331B1 discloses a method and kit for enhancing the natural fertility process. The kit includes a vaginal douche that is used prior to intercourse to enhance the sperm transportation and sustaining properties of the cervical mucus. The douche contains a balanced electrolyte solution, polysaccharides, and pH buffers. The kit also includes nutraceuticals specifically formulated for both the male and female which include amino acids, minerals, vitamins, herbs, Phytoestrogens, and antioxidants along with a specified dosing regimen. A basal body temperature thermometer and chart is

provided with instructions to confirm when and if ovulation will/did occur. Commercially available urinary chemical reagent strips are provided with instructions so as to predict/confirm if and when ovulation will occur. A lubricating medium will also be provided and utilised at the time of intercourse which is no spermicidal and which contains polysaccharides which influence natural sperm motility. A detailed instruction book regarding the method and practice is provided along with dietary and lifestyle recommendations which have been shown to affect natural fertility.

US20100144030Al discloses methods and apparatus to separate X or Y-chromosome bearing sperm cells in a population by first placing the population of sperm cells at physiological pH environment, and simultaneously contacting the population of sperm cells with one or more additional sub- environments with different pH values. The exposure allows mobile sperm cells bearing X or Y-chromosome to migrate to the different pH sub-environments, wherein each cell only exposed or come in contact with one pH sub-environment. Finally, the collecting X or Y-chromosome enriched population of sperm cells is performed.

AU2016412421A1 discloses a novel compressed tablet composition for helping to living birth to female child. The effectiveness of the drug depends on two theories, "Thickness of the egg coat" and "Cell Fragility". The first theory proves that the egg coat differs in thickness from one woman to another; being the major factor in determining the sex of the baby. The second theory indicates the factors of strength, weakness and fragility of living cells in general and of corona radiate in

particular Hingorani V., Shroff G., in their article titled as "Natural Sex Selection for Safe Motherhood and as a Solution for Population Control", published in the International Journal of Gynecology and Obstetrics, 1995, discloses "For Safe Motherhood wanted children should be of desired sex. As Y sperm have a shorter lite span and migrate faster, if coitus occurs before ovulation, sperm must wait in the tube for the ovum to arrive. By the time the ovum arrives, Y sperm have died and X sperm fertilize the ovum, resulting in a baby girl. If coitus takes place after ovulation when the ovum is waiting in the tube, the faster migrating Y sperm fertilizer the ovum resulting in a baby boy. Eighty women wishing to test this hypothesis by basal body temperature and ultrasound were recruited. Correct results have so far been obtained in 97%. This theory can be used for Safe Motherhood, for population control and to eliminate sex-linked genetic disorders. It can also prevent both female foeticide and infanticide in some cultures."

Lorrain, Jin an article titled as "Pre-Conceptional Sex Selection", published in the International Journal Gynecology and Obstetrics, 1975, discloses postconceptional and preconception methods of selecting fetal sex. Among the preconception methods presented are treatment of the sperm to isolate either the X or the Y chromosome, timing of insemination and the effect of ionic concentrations in the woman's body as controlled by the dietary intake of minerals. The authors studied 281 couples, 21 of whom were later excluded, who adhered to a diet specific in its amounts of calcium, magnesium, sodium and potassium. This dietary method of preconceptional selection of fetal sex resulted in the anticipated outcome in about 80% of the cases.

Stolkowski, J., Choukroun J., in their article titled as "Preconception Selection of Sex in Man", published in Israel Journal of Medical Sciences, 1981, disclose that the determination of sex is influenced by ionic factors. In man, ionic imbalance is responsible for the sex ratio in at least

80% of cases, the possible mechanism being one of selective fertilization. These facts constitute the scientific basis for the medicodietary method of selecting sex. The intervention of ions in ovarian metabolism is obtained by controlling the diet of the woman, the decisive factor being the ratio of K++ Na + to C a2++Mg2+ in the daily diet. High values of this ratio lead to boys, and low values to girls. Using this method since 1970 in 47 births, only 7 of them failed to produce the expected sex. The interactions and the causes of failure are analysed.

Zarutskie P.W., Muller C.H. Magone M., Soules, M.R., in their article titled as "The Clinical Relevance of Sex Selection Techniques", Fertility and Sterility, 1989, discloses that clinical and laboratory attempts to alter the sex ratio require more complete and thorough study. Improved identification of Y- bearing sperm through chromosome evaluation rather than by F-body identification is critical to provide a more precise definition. The tentative conclusions stated below are based on an assessment of literature from which it is generally difficult to draw conclusions: 1. The timing of intercourse in relation to ovulation and subsequent fertilisation appears to influence the sex ratio. More females are conceived when coitus occurs relatively close to ovulation, and more males are conceived when the sperm or egg is in the reproductive tract for a relatively longer time before conception. The influence of coital timing on the sex ratio is overall quite subtle and is not a practical method to alter the sex ratio for individual couples. 2. The use of ovulation-inducing medications slightly favors female offspring. A decrease in sex ratio of 5% to 10% has been shown in multiple studies. Artificial insemination with fresh donor or homologous spermatozoa results in more male births with a reported 7% to 10% increase in the sex ratio. It appears with induction combined that ovulation artificial insemination cancels the respective influences of each on the sex ratio. 4. Sperm separation techniques using albumin (for selection of Y- bearing sperm) or Sephadex column filtration (for selection of X-bearing sperm) are the only techniques that have been reported to alter the sex ratio to a degree that is clinically relevant. Although clinical birth data are just beginning to accumulate, these methods appear to have a 70% to 80% success for selection of assumed Y-bearing sperm and a 75% to 80% success for selection of assumed X-bearing sperm. The validity of these results will remain questionable until fully detailed accounts are published and successfully repeated. Free-flow electrophoresis appears to achieve significant separation; however, the depressed post procedure spermatozoa motility presently limits the usefulness of this procedure. 5. There is a potential to combine clinical and laboratory methods to maximize the efficiency of sex selection for interested couples. Modern methods to identify ovulation (e.g., urinary LH kits, ultrasonography) may help the timing of coitus for sex selection. Clomiphene citrate may enhance female sex preselection when Sephadex column filtration is also employed. 6. The priority of sex preselection in terms of medical, social, and demographic consideration remains to be determined. The avoidance of sex-linked genetic disorders is a reasonable and desirable goal.

An article published in 2013, (https://www.indiaparentmagazine.org/article/amazing- discovery-women-have- alternating-boy-girl-boy-girl-type- menstrual-cycles.php) titled: Amazing discovery: women have alternating boy-girl-boy-girl type menstrual cycles, which discloses several discoveries in women have led us to develop unique PreGender pre-conception urine test to guide couples to conceive in specific cycle to get a baby boy or girl. Days of keep-trying are over.

An article (https://www.babycenter.in/a549359/choosing- your-babys-sex-the- folklore) discloses you're said to be more likely to conceive a girl if...

You have sex earlier on in your cycle, a few days before ovulation. This is because female sperm are thought to be stronger and therefore last longe than male sperm, who will die off before reaching the egg.

- Your husband reaches orgasm before you.

- You have sex frequently to lower your husband's sperm count, and so increase the chances of the female sperm reaching the egg first.
- You keep penetration shallow.
- You stop having unprotected sex four to five days before ovulation, to minimize the chances of the male sperm reaching the egg first.
- Your husband keeps his genitals warm by wearing close- fitting underwear and tight trousers (although this isn't likely to do his general fertility any good!).
- You suggested the love-making.
- You make love in the afternoon.
- You make love on even days of the month.
- You put a wooden spoon under your bed and a pink ribbon under your pillow.
- You drink plenty of milk and eat dairy products such as cheese and curd, salty foods, rice, pasta, certain vegetables, mineral water, limited amounts of meat and potatoes, but avoid wine and beer, fresh fruit, spinach, tomatoes and mushrooms, chocolate, coffee and tea.

**You're said to be more likely to conceive a boy if...**

- You have sex on the day of ovulation, as male sperm are thought to swim faster and reach the egg first.

- You reach orgasm before your husband, as this releases an alkaline fluid, thought to be more male-sperm friendly than the vagina's natural acidity.
- You have deep penetration during sex, such as from behind (doggy style).
- Your husband has a high sperm count. This is because male sperm are not as strong as female sperm, and so the higher the count, the more chance there is of a male sperm reaching the egg first.
- You avoid sex for a week before ovulation and then only have sex once on ovulation day, to keep the sperm count high.
- Your husband suggested the love-making.
- You make love at night.
- You make love on odd days of the month.
- Your husband keeps his genitals cool by wearing boxer shorts and loose-fitting trousers.
- You eat sweet food, plenty of meat, fish, white flour (maida), pasta, fresh fruit, certain vegetables, but avoid milk and dairy products, such as curd and cheese, nuts, chocolate, shellfish and wholemeal bread.

An article (https:// pubmed. ncbi. nlm. nih. gov/449885/) discloses that the proportion 10 of male babies was significantly higher (65.5 +/- 3.9 per cent, mean +/- S.D.) in COPYRIGHT OFF he offspring of women who resumed intercourse two days after ovulation. This NEW DELHI No-L- 130622 roportion tended to be lower on or near the day of ovulation than on the previous one or two days. These results, which were consistent in different demographic subgroups, demonstrate that insemination on different days of the menstrual cycle does lead to variations in sex ratio. Couples should be cautioned against attempting to conceive a boy by delaying intercourse until after ovulation, until further research has established whether delayed fertilisation causes birth defects.

An article (https://www.disabled-world.com/calculators- charts/baby.php) discloses "Various ways to try, including the Shettles Method, to conceive a boy or girl baby, includes baby gender predictor calculator. Until now, there has not yet been any scientific proof and recognition of the most effective methods in determining baby's sex before conception. Conception is most likely to happen if sex is performed prior to ovulation, and timing plays a large role in successful conception."

1. **The most important aspect of all is timing of intercourse during the monthly cycle.**

The closer to ovulation (Ovulation calculator) you have sex, the better the chances have a boy, because the y-sperms are faster and tend to get to the egg first. If you have sex 3 days or more before ovulation, the better your chances to conceive a girl, because the weaker y-sperms tend to die sooner and the x-sperms will be available in greater quantity whenever the egg is released. On the other hand, having sex from 2 days before ovulation, through a few days after ovulation, is better for conceiving a boy. Around the 2-day point, 48 hours before ovulation, seems to be the 50/50 mark.

**2. The pH of the women's tract is also very important.**

A more acidic environment favors girls, since it will kill the weaker y-sperms first, leaving a greater quantity of x- sperms available to fertilizer the egg. On the other hand, a more alkaline environment favors boys.

Shettles recommends a douche of water and vinegar (acid) immediately before intercourse to favor a girl; a douche of water and baking soda (alkaline) will help for a boy. (Don't try this without reading Shettles! You have to dilute the douches properly, according to his formula, or they won't help and might hurt you.)

**Note: Some women are naturally very acidic and have a hard time conceiving boys.**

**3. Position of intercourse and depth of penetration are important, partly because of pH.**

The closer to the entrance to the vagina, the more acidic the women's tract is. Also, deep penetration places the sperm closer to the egg, and gives those aggressive boy sperms a head start. So, a shallow penetration will favor girls - and deeper will favor boys. Shettles recommends the missionary-position for a girl, and rear-entry (doggy-style) for a boy.

**4. Women's orgasms can also be important.**

It also has to do with pH. When a woman has an orgasm, the body releases a substance that makes the environment more alkaline, favoring boys. He recommends no orgasms when trying for girls!

**5. The sperm count is another factor.**

Obviously, a low sperm count to begin with doesn't favor either sex. But a high sperm count favors boys. Shettles recommends three things:

a. When trying for a boy, don't have sex for 3-4 days before you reach the target date a day or two before ovulation! For girls, have sex every day from day = 1 or day
   = 5 ("cleaner") and stop 3 days before ovulation.
b. Shettles recommends that for boys, the man wear loose underwear only, that is, men who usually wear briefs or other tight underwear should switch to boxers.

The idea is the same as wearing boxers to increase overall fertility, the testicles need cooler temperatures for sperms to survive, and the Y-sperms, since they are helped more than the X-sperms by this method. However, Shettles does NOT recommend the opposite, that men wear briefs for a girl, this will just decrease overall fertility.

It is a well-known fact that gender is determined by the presence of two 'X' chromosomes (XX) in female and one 'X' chromosome and one 'Y' chromosome in male. The sex cells i.e. the sperm and ovum are formed by meiotic division of diploid germinal cells. Ovum is produced in the ovary from diploid female germinal cells (containing 44 autosomes and 2 'X'). So only one type of ovum is produced containing 23 autosomes and 1' * X' chromosome in the ovary. The sperm is produced in the testes from diploid male germinal cells containing 44 autosomes and 1^* X' chromosome and 1^* y' chromosome. Hence, two types of sperms are produced in the testes. One type containing 23 autosomes and I 'X' chromosome and the other type containing 23 autosomes and I 'Y' chromosome. As these two types sperms are produced in equal numbers so there is a 50-50 chance of conceiving either gender. After fertilisation an XX zygote will develop into a female child and an XY zygote will develop into a male child.

The existing processes have not taken into consideration many key factors involved in the process of fertilisation of a sperm with an ovum that influence conception of a child of desired gender, which may result in un intended conceptions.

The present inventors have identified several key factors that can be manipulated to increase the chances of fertilisation by an "X" carrying sperm, thereby increasing the potential of conceiving a female child, or alternatively to increase the chances of fertilisation by a "Y" carrying sperm, thereby increasing the potential of conceiving a male child.

# OBJECTS OF THE WORK

Some of the objects of the present work, which at least one embodiment herein, satieties are as follows-

An object of the present work is to ameliorate one or more problems of the prior art or to at least provide a useful alternative.

The primary objective of the present work is to provide a method of reproduction by selective fertilization of gametes in humans.

Another objective of the present work is to provide a method to produce a child with a desired gender, and to create a balance in the family as well as in the society.

A further objective of the present work is to control the growth of population, eradicate female foeticide, poverty, property division disputes by following the principle of family planning and to bring gender balance in the society as well as family "Hum Do Hamare Do Ek Beta Ek Beti Ho" i.e. "We -

Two, Our Two One Son, One Daughter"

Other objectives, features and advantages will become apparent to those skilled in the art from the detailed description and the appended claims.

# SUMMARY OF THE WORK

The present work provides a method of reproduction by selective fertilisation of gametes in humans. To plan a child in this method, the woman on the 8th day of the menstrual cycle (MC) undergoes Hysterosalpingogram (HSG) Test to know the status of the oviduct. If the oviducts are normal then the woman undergoes another test i.e. Follicular Monitoring Test (FMT) every day from 9th day to 14th day of the MC to observe the enlargement of ovary and rupturing of the follicle is going on in which side ovary i.e. in the right-side ovary or in the left side ovary. Rupturing of follicle is also necessary to observe during the FMT test.

Wherein based on the HSG Test on the 8th day of the MC, if the status of both oviducts found not to be normal, this means they are not functioning normally, oviducts to normalcy if possible. Based on the advice of the gynecologist if required the woman can check the status of her oviduct after the preliminary treatment from 8th day until 11th day of her MC. If the status of the oviduct is not normal up to the 11th day of MC, then she waits for the next MC or wait until the treatment is over or wait until the oviducts become normal. If the oviducts do not become normal even after treatment, the couple may move for in-vitro fertilisation (IVF) in the desire of a child.

During FMT, (which start from 9th day of MC) on or after the 12th day, but until or before the 14th day of the MC, when the required enlargement of ovary and rupturing of the follicle is observed, the couple plans for intercourse. Enlargement of the left side ovary will lead to the conception of a female child, whereas, enlargement of the right side ovary will lead to the conception of a male child. Another aspect of the present work is the use of a sideways elevated bed to facilitate the flow of semen from the uterus to the oviduct of the desired side of ovary.

# DETAILED DESCRIPTION OF THE WORK

The preferred embodiments of the present work will be described in detail with the following disclosure and examples. The foregoing general description and the following detailed description are provided to illustrate only some embodiments of the present work and not to limit the scope of the present work. The work is capable of other embodiments and can be carried out or practiced in various other ways.

Unless otherwise specified, all the technical and scientific terms used herein have the same meaning as is generally understood by a person skilled in the art pertaining to the present work.

Headings are used solely for organisational purposes, and are not intended to limit the work in any way.

The use of the singular includes the plural unless specifically stated otherwise. As used herein, the singular forms "a," "an" and "the" are intended to include the plural forms as well. The use of "or" means "and/or" unless stated otherwise.

As used herein, the terms "comprises" and/or "comprising" specify the presence of the stated features, integers, steps, operations, elements, and/or components, but do not preclude the presence or addition of one or more other features, integers, steps, operations, elements, components, and/or groups thereof. Furthermore, to the extent that the terms "includes," "having," "has," "with," "composed," "comprised" or variants thereof are used in either the detailed description or the claims, such terms are intended to be inclusive in a manner similar to the term "comprising."

As used herein, ranges and amounts can be expressed as "about" a particular value or range. "About" is intended to also include the exact amount. Hence "about 5 percent" means "about 5 percent" and also "5 percent." "About" means within typical experimental error for the application or purpose intended.

It is to be understood that wherein a numerical range is recited, it includes all values within that range, and all narrower ranges within that range, whether specifically recited or not.

Reference throughout this specification to "one embodiment," "an embodiment," "one example," or "an example" means that a particular feature, structure, or characteristic described in connection with the embodiment or example is included in at least one embodiment of the present work. Thus, appearances of the phrases "in one embodiment," "in an embodiment," "one example," or "an 10 example" in various places throughout this specification are not necessarily all

Terring to the same embodiment or example. Furthermore, the particular Aare's, structures, or characteristics may be combined in any suitable and/or sub-combinations in one or more embodiments or examples. In addition, it should be appreciated that if any figures are provided herewith, they are for explanation purposes to persons ordinarily skilled in the art and that the drawings of them are not necessarily drawn to scale.

In this specification, certain aspects of one embodiment include process steps and/or operations and/or instructions described herein for illustrative purposes in a particular order and/or grouping. However, the particular order and/or grouping shown and discussed herein are illustrative only and not limiting. Those of skill in the art will recognize that other orders and/or grouping of the process steps and/or operations and/or instructions are possible and, in some embodiments, one or more of the process steps and/or operations and/or instructions discussed above can be combined and/or deleted. In addition, portions of one or more of the process steps and/or operations and/or instructions can be re-grouped as portions of one or more other of the process steps and/or operations and/or instructions discussed herein. Consequently, the particular order and/or grouping of the process steps and/or operations and/or instructions discussed herein do not limit

The present work provides a method of reproduction by selective fertilisation of gametes in human for a woman to conceive a child with a desired gender by influencing certain factors in the process of fertilisation. The method includes several steps as provided below in brief and described further in a detailed manner.

The method helps a couple to follow certain systematic procedures involved in the process of fertilisation to conceive a child of desired gender.

The steps of this method are simple to follow and they greatly influence the conditions of conceiving a child of desired gender. When the steps are performed (methodical and disciplined manner, the success rate of conceiving a child of a gender increases by manifolds.

The knowledge of the ovulation from a particular side of ovary (right side or left side) in a specific menstrual cycle (MC) plays a vital role to perform the first step of the method of the present work.

It is our finding and is well known to me that, the ovum produced from right side ovary attracts Y chromosome bearing sperm and it is repulsive to the X chromosome bearing sperms. In the same manner, ovum produced from left side ovary attracts X chromosome bearing sperms and it is repulsive to the Y chromosome bearing sperms. The reason behind this selective nature of the ovum produced from the right side ovary and the left side ovary lies in the secretion of hormones and the flow of electrolytes, which results in different level of activation of the left side or the right side of the female body in alternate menstruation cycles (MC).

In order to know the time of ovulation and the side of the ovary from which the ovulation is going to happen in a particular menstrual cycle, it is important that the woman has a good knowledge of the length of her menstrual cycle. The length of a normal menstrual cycle is 28 days. However, some women have their MC length as short as 21 days and as long as 40 days. In such case women should go to the doctor to regulate it. But the length. of MC of an individual woman remains. consistent from one cycle to the next cycle. The ovulation generally happens on the day that is the midpoint of the MC. For example, in a 28 day MC, ovulation typically occurs about 14 day before the start of the next MC. But in most women ovulation occurs before four days of the midpoint of the MC or four days after the midpoint of the MC. It is important that the woman has a good understanding of this concept.

The status of the oviduct of the woman is observed on the day that is 8 days before the midpoint day of the menstrual cycle (MC) through HSG Test. If the oviducts are normal then the woman undergoes another test procedure i.e. follicular Monitoring Test (FMT) continuously once a day from the day that is five days before the midpoint day of the menstrual cycle (MC) to the midpoint day of the MC to observe the enlargement of ovary and rupturing of the follicle is going on in which side ovary i.e. in the right side ovary or in the left side ovary.

Wherein based on the HSG Test on the day that is 8th days before the midpoint day of the menstrual cycle (MC), if the status of oviducts are found not to be normal, this means they are not functioning normally, then the woman visits a gynecologist to get the required treatment to bring the oviducts to normalcy if possible. Based on the advice of the gynecologist if required the woman can check the status of her oviduct after the preliminary treatment from the day that is 6 days before the midpoint day of the menstrual cycle (MC) until the day that is 3 days before the midpoint day of the menstrual cycle (MC). If the status of the oviduct is not normal up to the day that is 3 days before the midpoint day of the menstrual cycle (MC), then she waits for the next MC or wait until the treatment is over or wait until the oviducts become normal. If the oviducts do not become normal even after treatment, the couple may move for in-vitro fertilisation (IVF) in the desire of a child.

From the regular observation of the report of FMT from the day that is 5 days before the midpoint day of the menstrual cycle (MC) till the day that is two days before the midpoint day of the menstrual cycle (MC), if it is found that the left side ovary is enlarged, which means ovulation will occur from the left side ovary.

If the couple is eager to conceive a female child, then they perform intercourse on the day that is 2 days before the midpoint day of the menstrual cycle (MC) and continue it every day until the midpoint day of the MC. If the couple is not eager to have a female child then they wait for the next cycle as ovulation happens alternately from left and right side ovary every month. When from the day that is 2 days before the midpoint day of the menstrual cycle (MC), report of the FMT enlargement of the right side ovary and rupturing of the follicle is observed, which means ovulation will occur from the right side ovary and if the couple is eager to conceive a male child then they perform intercourse on the day that is two days before the midpoint day of the menstrual cycle (MC) and continue it every day until the midpoint day of the MC. If the couple is not eager to have a male child, then they wait for the next MC.

On or after the day that is 2 days before the midpoint day of the menstrual cycle (MC), but until or before the midpoint day of the MC, when the required enlargement of ovary and rupturing of the follicle of the desired side is observed from FMT, the couple plan to have intercourse from the day that is 2 days before the midpoint day of the menstrual cycle (MC) day till midpoint day of the MC by taking guided precautions and following specific steps during and after intercourse in a stepwise manner, which are given below.

The couple take light meal so as to keep their stomachs 50% to 75% full to avoid indigestion due to the requirement of the process to sleep on a single side of the body for long time after intercourse, and the woman finishes urination to have her

urinary bladder empty before going to bed. The length of the bed is 20% or more longer than the length of the taller person among the woman and the man. The couple go to bed early so that they can spend some good quality time in love making and remain in a happy mood all through the process and to get sufficient time for the fertilisation of the ovum by the sperm.

In an aspect the woman and the man at the same time go to the bed immediately after the woman urinates.

In another aspect, the man is already present on the bed when the woman goes to the bed immediately after urination.

In another aspect, the man and the woman both urinate to have their urinary bladders empty, and go to the bed together immediately after urination.

In an embodiment of the work, while performing intercourse, the woman keeps a pillow below her hip to allow the flow of semen towards the oviduct from vagina successfully in enough quantity. This elevated position of the woman also helps in the successful flow of semen in enough quantity even if there is low sperm count. Once ejaculation is completed sexual intercourse is stopped to prevent the dislodging of any of the ejaculate from the vagina. The woman avoid urination or bowel movement after intercourse is completed to prevent the expulsion of the ejaculate from the vagina. Soon after ejaculation the woman turns towards her left side or right side according to the plan of conceiving a female child or male child and remain in that position to facilitate the movement of maximum semen towards the uterus and simultaneously stop the loss of semen from the vagina.

The woman lies by keeping her left side on the bed if the couple have opted to conceive a female child after observing the report of the FMT. Some kind of obstructive material may be kept on the back of the woman's body so as to prevent her from changing her side to the right while sleeping. If the couple have opted to conceive a male child after observing the report of FMT, then after ejaculation the woman lies on the bed by keeping her right side on the bed. Some kind of obstructive material may be kept on the back of her body to prevent her to change her side to the left while sleeping. This particular type of sleeping position of the woman after ejaculation aids in the movement of the semen to the oviduct where fertilisation will Occur.

In an alternative embodiment of the present work, instead of keeping any obstructive material on the back of the woman, the couple do intercourse on a ways, elevated bed, wherein the length of the bed is 20% or more longer than of the taller person among the woman and the man. If the couple have planned to conceive a female child, the woman after ejaculation by the man, sleeps by keeping the left side of her body down on the right side of elevated bed which will prevent her movement towards right while in sleep. Similarly if the couple have planned to conceive a male child, the woman sleeps by keeping the right side of her body down, on the left side of elevated bed which will prevent her movement towards the left side during sleep.

The woman sleeps in the required kind of position after ejaculation according to the plan of conceiving a female child or a male child for (at least) 7 to 8 hours without any disturbance.

In order to have a male child or a female child a method has

been devised. The method is performed in a stepwise manner.

**Examples:**

The present work will now be explained in further detail by the following examples. These examples are illustrative of certain embodiments of the work without limiting the scope of the present work.

**Example 1**

A woman has a typical 28 day MC. On the 8th day of her MC the woman underwent Hysterosalpingogram (HSG) Test to know the status of the oviduct, and found that the oviducts were normal. Then, the woman underwent Follicular Monitoring Test (FMT) on the 9th day of the MC, and found there was no enlargement of any ovary. The woman underwent FMT on the 10th day of the MC, and found there was no enlargement of right ovary. It remains constant in size The woman underwent FMT on the 11thday of the MC, and found there was no enlargement of right ovary. But it shows enlargement in left ovary. The woman underwent FMT on the 12thday of the MC, and found that there was enlargement of her left side ovary and rupturing of the follicle, which meant that ovulation occurred from the left side ovary. The couple eager to have a male child, so they stopped the plan in that MC and wait for next MC.

**Example 2**

A woman has a typical or normal 28 day MC. On the 8th day of her MC the woman underwent Hysterosalpingogram (HSG) Test to know the status of the oviduct, and found that the oviducts were normal. Then, the woman underwent Follicular Monitoring Test (FMT) on the 9th day of the MC, and found there was no enlargement of any ovary. The woman underwent FMT on the 10th day of the MC, and found there was no enlargement of left ovary. But it shows enlargement in right ovary. The woman underwent FMT on the 11th day of the MC, and found through FMT that there was enlargement of her right-side ovary and rupturing of the follicle, which meant that ovulation occurred from the right-side ovary and will provide male child.

On the evening of the 12th day at 7 pm, the woman and her man partner were in a happy mood and they took a light meal so as to keep their stomachs 50% to 75% full to avoid indigestion due to the requirement of the process to sleep on a single side of the body for long time after intercourse, and the woman finished her "urination before going to bed. The length of the bed was 6.5 feet long and 5.5 feet vide. The couple went to bed at 8.30 pm, and a pillow was kept below the woman's hip, and they started intercourse in a normal intercourse position woman lying at the bottom with belly up, and the man performing the intercourse with belly down on the woman. After ejaculation is completed, sexual intercourse was stopped to prevent the dislodging of any of the ejaculate from the vagina.

Soon after ejaculation the woman turned towards her right side and remained in that position for 7 to 8 hours without any disturbance.

The same procedure they continued on the 13th day and on the 14th day too if possible.

She did not get her next period i.e. she did not menstruate as she regularly does. She went for the pregnancy test by using a pregnancy kit, and it was found that she was pregnant. They confirmed the same on the next day with another kit to reconfirm. And the pregnancy was confirmed.

The couple went for checkups with the gynecologist.

After 276 days of the Last menstrual period (LMP) the woman gave birth to a male child.

**Example 3**

A woman has a typical 28-day MC. On the 8th day of her MC the woman underwent Hysterosalpingogram (HSG) Test to know the status of the oviduct, and found that the oviducts were not normal. She met a gynecologist, and got the required treatment to bring the oviducts to normalcy if possible. The status of the oviduct was not normal up to the 11th day of MC. So she waited for the next MC or wait until the treatment is over or wait until the oviducts become normal. If the oviducts do not become normal even after treatment, the couple may move for in- vitro fertilisation (IVF) with the desire of a child.

**Advantages:**

The method of the present work has the following major advantages.

Solution to the problem of population explosion as people may have many female children for the need of single male child.

Maintain gender ratio, Reduction or eradication of gender crimes, foeticide, property disputes in the families and huge pendency of civil suits in the courts, continuation of ancestral chain, getting male or female child without going for unethical gender determination (in certain countries including India) tests, and resulting again unethical foeticide. Fertilisation despite low sperm count

Although the present work is described in terms of certain preferred embodiments, it is to be understood that they have been presented by way of example, and not limitation. Thus, the present work should not be limited by any of the above- described exemplary embodiments, but should be defined only in accordance with the following claims and their equivalents.

# CLAIMS

**We claim:**

1. A method of reproduction by selective fertilisation of gametes in humans, for a woman to conceive a child with a desired gender by influencing certain factors in the process of fertilisation, wherein the method comprising the steps of:

- Observing the status of the oviduct of the woman on the 8th day of the menstrual cycle (MC) through HSG Test;
- When the status of the oviducts are found to be normal the woman undergoing
- Follicular Monitoring Test (FMT) once a day from the ninth day of the MC to fourteenth day of the MC upto rupturing to observe the enlargement of left or right side ovary, and rupturing of the follicle;
- The woman planning for vaginal intercourse with a man between the twelfth day until the fourteenth day of the MC when enlargement of an ovary and rupturing of the follicle is observed from the FMT;
- Providing a bed for the intercourse, wherein the length of the bed is 20% or more longer than the length of the taller person among the woman and the man;
- The woman and the man each taking a light meal so as to have their stomachs 50% to 75% full;

- The woman doing urination to have her urinary bladder empty;
- Immediately after urination, the woman and the man going to the bed within 30 minutes to 2 hours of taking the light meal;
- the woman sleeping with her body aligned on the longitudinal side of the bed with her belly up and back down position;
- the woman and the man doing the intercourse on the bed;
- the man ejaculating semen deepest possible into the woman's vagina;
- immediately after said ejaculation, the woman turning to her left side down position if a female child is desired to be conceived, or turning to her right side down position if a male child is desired to be conceived; and the woman sleeping for seven to eight hours in said left side down position or said right side down position without any disturbance.

2. The method as claimed in claim 1, wherein the couple desiring to have a female child planning for intercourse form the twelfth day until the fourteenth day of the MC when the enlargement of the left side ovary and rupturing of the follicle is observed from the FMT,

3. The method as claimed in claim 1, wherein the woman and he man at the same time go to the bed.
4. The method as claimed in claim 1, wherein the man is already present on the bed, when the woman goes to the bed immediately after urination.
5. The method as claimed in claim 1, wherein the couple desiring to have a male Child planning for intercourse form the MC when the enlargement of the right side ovary and rupturing of the follicle is observed from the FMT.
6. The method as claimed in claim 1, wherein the woman performs vaginal intercourse with a man, every day from the twelfth day until the fourteenth day of the MC when enlargement of an ovary and rupturing of the follicle is observed from the FMT.
7. The method as claimed in claim 1, wherein the woman performs vaginal intercourse with a man, more than one time every day from the twelfth day until the fourteenth day of the MC when enlargement of an ovary and rupturing of the follicle is observed from the FMT.
8. The method as claimed in claim 1, wherein the intercourse is done at any time in a day, preferably after a meal time.
9. The method as claimed in claim 1, wherein the intercourse is done after the dinner.

10. The method as claimed in claim 1, wherein the intercourse is done after the dinner, wherein the dinner is completed earlier in the evening.

11. The method as claimed in claim 1, wherein the intercourse is done after the lunch.

12. The method as claimed in claim I, wherein the intercourse is done after the breakfast.

13. The method as claimed in claim 1, wherein the intercourse is done after the breakfast, wherein the breakfast is completed earlier in the morning.

14. The method as claimed in claim 1, wherein an obstructive material is kept on the back side of the woman to prevent any sideways movement.

15. The method as claimed in claim 1, wherein a sideways elevated bed, wherein the top surface of the bed is formed in a sloping manner such that one side of the bed is elevated in a sloping manner in comparison to its opposite side.

16. The method as claimed in claim 15, wherein the couple desiring to have a female child use a right side elevated bed, and the woman after ejaculation, sleeps by keeping the left side of her body down on the right side of the right side elevated bed.

17. The method as claimed in claim 15, wherein the couple desiring to have a male child use a left side elevated bed, and the woman after said

ejaculation, sleeps by keeping the right side of her body down on the left side of the left side elevated bed.

18. A method of reproduction by selective fertilisation of gametes in humans, for a woman to conceive a child with a desired gender by influencing certain factors in the process of fertilisation, wherein the method comprising the steps of: observing the status of the oviduct of the woman on the day that is 8 days before the midpoint day of the menstrual cycle (MC) through HSG Test;

When the status of the oviducts are found to be normal the woman undergoing Follicular Monitoring Test (FMT) once a day from the day that is 5 days before the midpoint day of the menstrual cycle (MC) to observe the enlargement of left and right side ovary, and rupturing of the follicle; The woman planning for vaginal intercourse with a man between the day that is two days before the midpoint day of the menstrual cycle (MC) until the midpoint day of the MC when enlargement of an ovary and rupturing of the follicle is observed from the FMT; providing a bed for the intercourse, wherein the length of the bed is 20% or more longer than the length of the taller person among the woman and the man: the woman and the man each taking a light meal so as to have their stomachs 50% to 75% full; The woman doing urination to have her urinary bladder empty; immediately after urination, the woman and the man going to the bed within 30 minutes to 2 hours of taking the light meal; the woman sleeping with her body aligned on the longitudinal side of the bed her belly up and back down position. The woman and the man doing the intercourse on the bed. The man ejaculating semen deepest possible into the woman's vagina;

Immediately after said ejaculation, the woman turning to her left side down position if a female child is desired to be conceived, or turning to her right side down position if a male child is desired to be conceived; and the woman sleeping for seven to eight hours in said left side down position or said right side down position without any disturbance.

# SECRETS OF CHILD TECHNOLOGY

Matter on which copy right is provided by the copyright department of India

INVENTION DISCLOSURE FORM

## Section A

| AI. INVENTOR(S) | | | | |
|---|---|---|---|---|
| | NAME (FULL with expanded initials) | NATIONALITY | GENDE | MAILING ADDRESS WITH PIN CODE |
| 1 | SHIV RAM TIWARI | INDIAN | MALE | 15-B, PANCHVATI COLONY, PICNIC SPOT ROAD, KHURRAM NAGAR, MAHANAGAR, LUCKNOW 226006, UTTAR |
| 2 | JAMVAN TI TIWARI | INDIAN | FEMAL | 15-B, PANCHVATI COLONY, PICNIC SPOT ROAD, KHURRAM NAGAR, MAHANAGAR, LUCKNOW 226006, UTTAR |

have her urinary bladder empty; immediately after urination, the woman and the man going to the bed within 30 minutes to 2 hours of taking the light meal; the woman sleeping with her body aligned on the longitudinal side of the bed her belly up and back down position. The woman and the man doing the intercourse on the bed. The man ejaculating semen deepest possible into the woman's vagina;

Immediately after said ejaculation, the woman turning to her left side down position if a female child is desired to be conceived, or turning to her right side down position if a male child is desired to be conceived; and the woman sleeping for seven to eight hours in said left side down position or said right side down position without any disturbance.

Matter on which copy right is provided by the copyright department of India

INVENTION DISCLOSURE FORM

## Section A

| AI. INVENTOR(S) | | | | |
|---|---|---|---|---|
| | NAME (FULL with expanded initials) | NATIONALITY | GENDE | MAILING ADDRESS WITH PIN CODE |
| 1 | SHIV RAM TIWARI | INDIAN | MALE | 15-B, PANCHVATI COLONY, PICNIC SPOT ROAD, KHURRAM NAGAR, MAHANAGAR, LUCKNOW 226006, UTTAR |
| 2 | JAMVAN TI TIWARI | INDIAN | FEMAL | 15-B, PANCHVATI COLONY, PICNIC SPOT ROAD, KHURRAM NAGAR, MAHANAGAR, LUCKNOW 226006, UTTAR |

| A2. APPLICANT(S | | | | |
|---|---|---|---|---|
| | NAME (FULL with expanded initials) | NATIONALIT | GENDE | MAILING ADDRESS WITH PIN CODE |
| 1 | SHIV RAM TIWARI | INDIAN | MALE | 15-B, PANCHVATI COLONY, PICNIC SPOT ROAD, KHURRAM NAGAR, MAHANAGAR, LUCKNOW 226006, UTTAR |
| 2 | JAMVAN TIWARI | INDIAN | FEMAL | 15-B, PANCHVATI COLONY, PICNIC SPOT ROAD, KHURRAM NAGAR, MAHANAGAR, LUCKNOW 226006, UTTAR |

## Section B

**B1. TITLE** (If you have it ready, else leave it.)

Innovation of Natural Bio-Mechanism of Reproduction by selective fertilization of gametes in human life

**B2. ABSTRACT** (If you have it ready, else leave it.)


In this respect I have involved two technological tests which are most important:

1. HSG-Hysterosalpingogram: By which we can know the status of oviduct or fallopian tube.
2. FMT-Follicular Monitoring Test: By which we can know the development of Ovum and its rupturing is normal or not.
3. Further one more technology is used i.e. an Elevated Bed. It should be one side elevated for/ to increase the probability of successful fertilization in a single process. This elevated bed directs the flow sperms towards the desired ovum through fallopian tube to give desired child male/female to make gender balance in society.
4. One more very important technology that already exist in female body itself is very specific protein found in outer corona layer of ovum. <u>This protein is responsible to attract the sperm for ovum as well as isolate them in X & Y sperm and allow for like insemination of ovum to produce XY Male Child or XX Female Child.</u>
5. This protein is discovered by some western scientist and they name it as PDILT which according

to them attracts the sperm towards ovum only for fertilization, but my assumption is that <u>this protein not only attracts the sperms but isolate them into X & Y from semen for like Inseminations for that ovum.</u>

**B3. LIMITATIONS OF THE EXISTING TECHNOLOGY** (Whatever you know, provide, else leave it.)

Please elaborate the problem being solved by your invention. Please specify any drawbacks in the Prior Existing knowledge/technology/product/process.

1. In females Both Fallopian Tubes should be normal in functioning, there should not be any blockage in them.
2. In females Ovulation should be in normal cycle with normal rupturing.
3. There should not be any type of cyst/obstacle in ovaries and also in uterus in females.
4. In males the sperm count should be normal.

**B4. RELEVANT PRIOR ART REFERENCES** (Whatever you know, provide, else leave it.) If you know, provide the Patent Numbers, or details of articles, or any other prior Art information.

**B5. NEW FEATURES OF THE INVENTION**

What are the novel aspects of your invention that need protection?

Describe technical difference between the conventional and available product/process and your solution. Please provide you how your solution is unique and different as compared with other available/known solutions to the same/similar problems.

1. To provide like child to the needy persons to balance the family as well as the society to save generations, to control populations to control foeticide, poverty, property division disputes by following "Hum Do Hamare Do-Ek Beta Ek Beti Ho".
2. Without knowing or applying the said technology people may have many female children for the need of single male child. In this way population and problem increases in family as well as in the society.
3. Many people in society are unknown of this technology to get like child. It is by chance they are getting male or female child
4. This whole concept depends upon the very specific protein present in outer most corona layer of ovum which isolates X & Y chromosomes wearing sperms from the semen for selective fertilization of the ovum of Left or Right side of the ovary.

**B6. DESCRIPTION OF THE INVENTION** (how the new features work to achieve the goal/objective)

Please detail the solution being provided by the invention to overcome the problems above. Please provide schematics diagram and its description if required.

Description of process for like child: During the menstrual cycle person should be alert for this concept that is child by planning and not by chance. For this on 8th day of MC, the lady should go for HSG (Hysterosalpingogram) Test at any trusted pathology and know the status of their oviduct. If they are normal it's good to proceed ahead. In this continuation from 9th day to 14th day the lady should go for FMT (Follicular Monitoring Test) to know the activity of the ovary and its rupturing also. If it is normal, then it's good to proceed ahead. Before rupturing the person should know the enlargement of size of the ovary through daily report of FMT on 12th day for further process.

If enlargement of ovary is in left side, the process will lead to the fertilization for female child and in case there is enlargement of ovary is in right side then it will lead to the fertilization for male child. Now couple should try on 12th night after MC with the precaution followed. For Example :-

1. They should take light meal at night to avoid indigestion to sleep towards the side for like child as mentioned above i.e. left side for female child and right side for male child.

2. They should go early to bed.
3. They should use elevated bed or use bricks or other material to elevate the bed by applying below both legs of the bed of opposite side in length to make slanting position towards right side for the flow of semen from uterus to the oviduct of right side ovary for 100% success of process in single attempt.
4. The lady should free from urination process before going to bed.
5. Female should keep a pillow below their abdomen to allow the flow of semen towards uterus from vagina successfully in enough quantity.
6. Now after taking all precaution they should enjoy the process of fertilization and just after ejaculation of semen, the female should tum towards right side and he should remain in same position for few minutes so that semen discharge should move maximum into the uterus otherwise it will come out of the vagina. Just for 100% success in single attempt said precaution is must. The slanting position of bed will help the female to remain in same position of right side. It will protect from any change from right side to left side. In this way, the female should sleep in same direction without any movement.

7. After this process they should continue their FMT till rupturing and can further repeat the same process on rupturing on 14th day of MC also.
8. By observing the FMT report of 12th day, if the person doesn't want to go for male child then the couple should not make efforts mentioned above and wait for next MC.
9. The FMT should continue till 14th day of MC to see the rupturing of ovum and avoid this pregnancy of MC on 12th and 14th day night.
10. Mostly rupturing occurs on 14th day of MC, if it comes on 28th day in cycle.
11. If the FMT shows enlargement in left ovary on 14th day of MC and the person wants male child then they should not make efforts towards fertilization on 12th as well as 14th day of MC.
12. They should avoid the process in this month and wait for next month of MC because functioning of ovary for ovulation will change next month as both the ovaries function to produce ovum alternatively.
13. Thus ovum of right ovary with X chromosome can produce male child after fertilization with Y chromosome sperms in oviduct which moved and settled in uterus for further development forming embryo and so on male child.

14. Here very specific contribution is of protein present in outer corona layer of ovum containing haploid X chromosome which attracts sperms from semen isolate them into haploid X & Y chromosomes wearing sperms and favours selective insemination by the right side ovum containing haploid X chromosomes for Y chromosomes bearing sperm only to form X Y Male embryo.

15. Same precaution should be taken in opposite direction for left side ovaries in case when female embryo/child is required.

# PHOTOGRAPHS OF THE RELATED CHILD

## TECHNOLOGY

### B.7 DRAWINGS (If any)

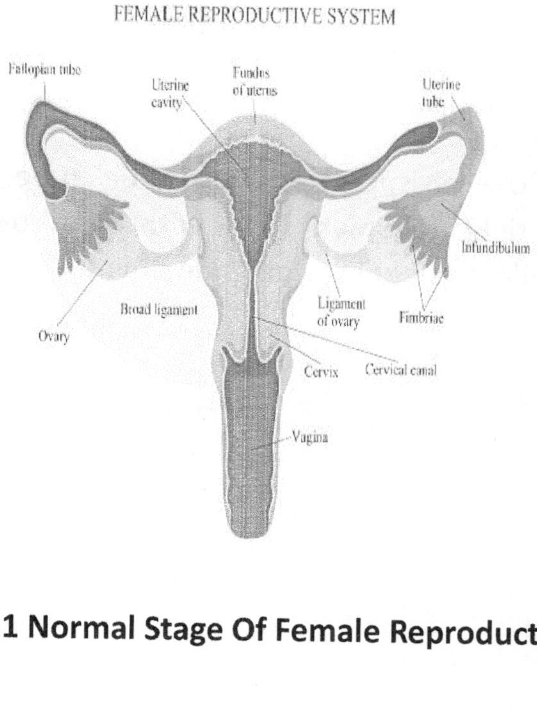


**Fig. 1 Normal Stage Of Female Reproductive Organ**

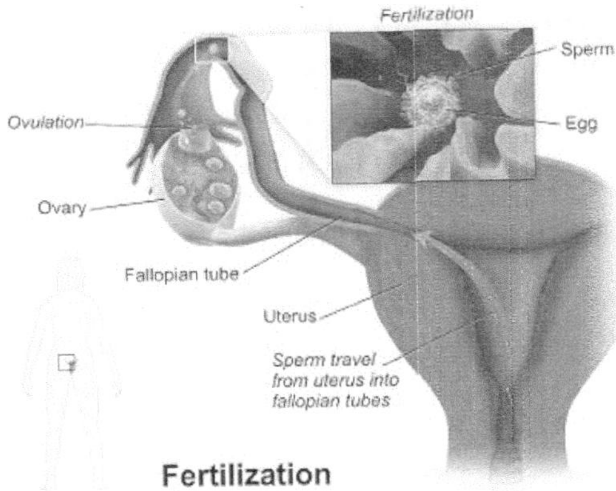


**Fig. Showing flow of sperm in right side tube for fertilization in right fallopian tube with right ovam provide male child by sleeping right side down**

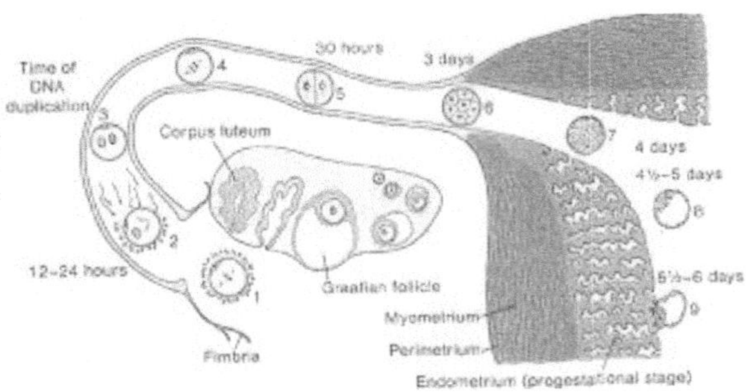


**Stages of Development of Embryo**

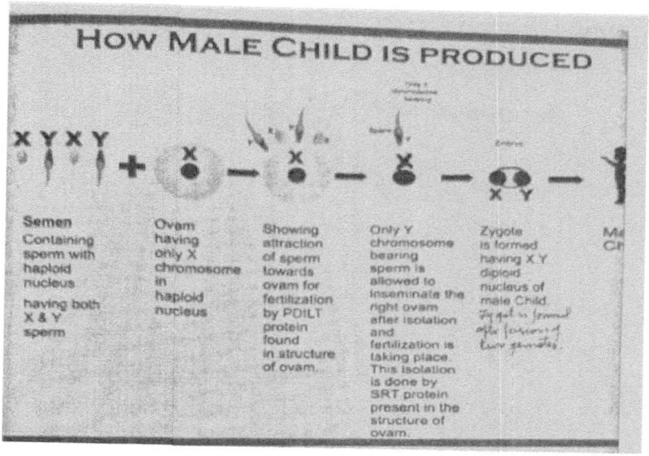


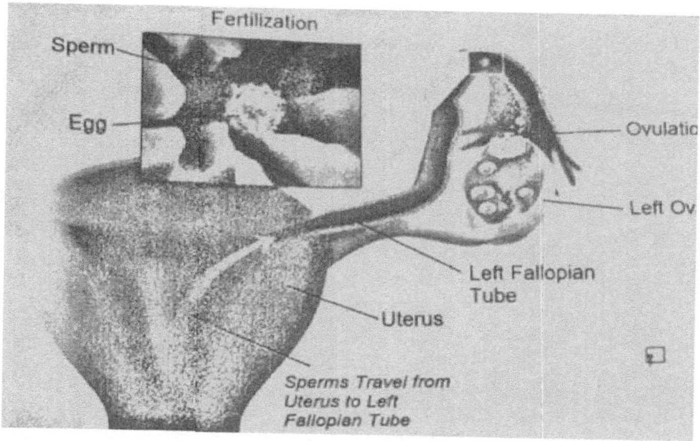


**Fig. Showing flow of sperm in left side tube for fertilization in left fallopian tube with left ovam to provide female child by sleeping left side dwon**

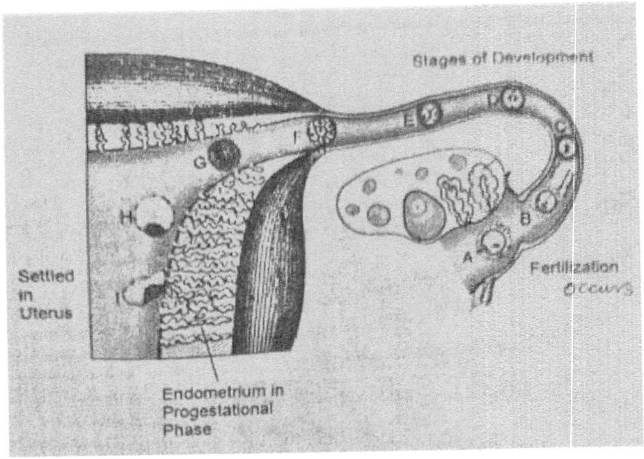


**Stages of Development of Embryo**

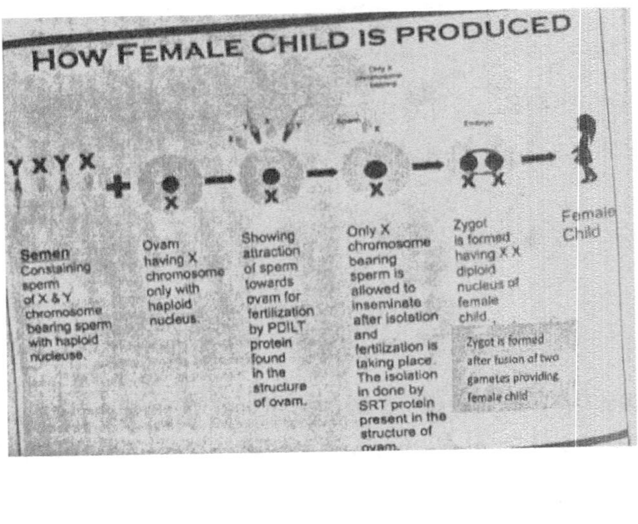

# DETAILS DESCRIPTION OF EACH DRAWING

## B8. A BRIEF DESCRIPTION OF EACH DRAWING

FIG 1 illustrates... internal parts of vagina, from uterus, right & left fallopian tube to right & left ovary

FIG 2A illustrates Movement of sperms from uterus towards right ovary

FIG. 2B illustrates... Stages of development from right ovary towards uterus

FIG 2C illustrates How Male Child is produced through right ovary

FIG. 3A illustrates Movement of sperms from uterus towards left ovary

FIG. 3B illustrates Stages of development from left ovary towards uterus

FIG 3C illustrates How Female Child is produced through left ovary

## B9. DETAILED DESCRIPTION OF EACH DRAWING

**As shown in Fig. 1,**

Picture of vaginal showing internal structure from Uterus to fallopian tube and ovaries.

**As shown in Fig. 2A & 2B,**

**The flow of semen/sperm from Vagina towards uterus and right oviduct facing downwards after ejaculation of semen for fertilization of ovum in right fallopian tube to produce male embryo of child.**

By taking all precautions for male embryo when process is going on among the couple on the bed. The flow of semen is controlled from vagina to uterus and right side of oviduct where haploid "X" chromosome bearing ovum is present for fertilization with isolated haploid "Y" chromosome bearing sperm. When the whole precaution is helpful to guide the flow of semen towards right-side of oviduct.

**As shown in Fig. 2C,**

**The corona Layer of Ovum getting activated containing very specific protein that attracts and Isolates "Y" chromosome bearing sperm from semen for selective insemination of ovum of right-side ovary to produce diploid "XY" male embryo of the child.**

It shows the role of very specific protein present in outer most layer of haploid ovum known as corona this protein attracts the sperm towards ovum as well as isolate them into "x" & "Y" chromosome bearing sperm. This isolated "Y" chromosome bearing sperm is only allowed to penetrate the ovum for Insemination known as "Fusion of Gametes" forming "XY" diploid embryo of male child which moves towards uterus and settled there for further division of cells and development into a Male Child.

**As shown in Fig. 3A & 3B,**

**The flow of semen/sperm from Vagina towards uterus and left oviduct facing downwards after ejaculation of semen for fertilization of ovum in left fallopian tube to produce female embryo of child.**

Similarly, by taking all precautions for male embryo when process is going on among the couple on the bed. The flow of semen is controlled from vagina to uterus and left-side of oviduct where haploid "X" chromosome bearing ovum is present for fertilization with isolated haploid "X" chromosome bearing sperm. When the whole precaution is helpful to guide the flow of semen towards left-side of oviduct.

**As shown in Fig. 3C,**

**The corona Layer of Ovum getting activated containing very specific protein that attracts and isolates "X" chromosome bearing sperm from semen for selective insemination of ovum of left-side ovary to produce diploid "XX" female embryo of the child.**

It shows the role of very specific protein present in outer most layer of haploid ovum known as corona this protein attracts the sperm towards ovum as well as isolate them into "X" & "Y" chromosome bearing sperm. This isolated "X" chromosome bearing sperm is only allowed to penetrate the ovum for insemination known as "Fusion of Garnetes" forming "XX" diploid embryo of female child which moves towards uterus and settled there for further division of cells and development into a Female Child.

## B10. ADVANTAGES

Please provide us the advantages of your solution? Please Compare the existing/conventional or solutions uncovered during the search under point 5. You may make a table or figures. Further you can provide us the economic potential or commercial applications for the technology.

The technology innovated by me is a noble work in the human life science in the world. It is very useful for birth of like child by the needy person in society as well as social balancing. In this way the technology is very successful in the interest of the nation to control burning problem of population i.e. to make population constant which is highly needed in developing countries like our India. Further to control foeticide, to uplift social status by having very balanced and complete happy family like "Hum Do Hamare Do-Ek Beta aur Ek Beti Ho". There will be least probability of property divisions and disputes in the families. To provide best possible education for children to strengthen the nation progress. Thus "Jab Hongi Uttam Santan Desh Banega Swayam Mahan" is motive of my life. One most important use of this concept is to balance the gender ratio in society as well as to fulfill the requirement of the needy couple.